MW00939786

CONSCIOUS HEALTH

Your Health Is Your Wealth

Davisson Edmond, M.D.

BALBOA.PRESS
A DIVISION OF HAY HOUSE

Copyright © 2021 Davisson Edmond, M.D.

All rights reserved. No part of this book may be used or reproduced by
any means, graphic, electronic, or mechanical, including photocopying,
recording, taping or by any information storage retrieval system
without the written permission of the author except in the case of
brief quotations embodied in critical articles and reviews.

Balboa Press books may be ordered through booksellers or by contacting:

Balboa Press
A Division of Hay House
1663 Liberty Drive
Bloomington, IN 47403
www.balboapress.com
844-682-1282

Because of the dynamic nature of the Internet, any web addresses or
links contained in this book may have changed since publication and
may no longer be valid. The views expressed in this work are solely those
of the author and do not necessarily reflect the views of the publisher,
and the publisher hereby disclaims any responsibility for them.

The author of this book does not dispense medical advice or prescribe the use
of any technique as a form of treatment for physical, emotional, or medical
problems without the advice of a physician, either directly or indirectly. The
intent of the author is only to offer information of a general nature to help
you in your quest for emotional and spiritual well-being. In the event you use
any of the information in this book for yourself, which is your constitutional
right, the author and the publisher assume no responsibility for your actions.

Any people depicted in stock imagery provided by Getty Images are
models, and such images are being used for illustrative purposes only.
Certain stock imagery © Getty Images.

Print information available on the last page.

ISBN: 978-1-9822-7114-5 (sc)
ISBN: 978-1-9822-7115-2 (e)

Library of Congress Control Number: 2021912953

Balboa Press rev. date: 06/25/2021

If you believe you should be responsible for your health and well-being, this book is for you. Dr. Edmond is a living example that you can practice what you preach. He lays out, in a simple and easy way to read, how to take care of your mind, body, and spirit.

Elie Ciril, MD

Your wealth is your health. This book is an interesting look into our most precious gift—our health—that we should take care of and cherish. Thanks, Dr. Edmond, to remind everyone that conscious health should be our key priority to a long-fulfilled existence.

Joseph Durandis, MD

To my family, my ultimate motivation in life, to my close friends for their unconditional love and support, and to those of you reading this book. I hope it restores awareness of your limitless potential.

CONTENTS

FOREWORD

The time has long-since come to shift our paradigm for how we regard and use the medical and wellness professions in creating and maintaining a healthy, vibrant, and disease-free lifestyle. The old Greek adage of healthy body/healthy mind, acknowledging an inextricable connection among the two, is even more true today as we are bombarded with all sorts of toxins ranging from environmental pollution, to radiation from our cellphones and computers, to just plain political noise that interferes with clarity of thought and healing states of mind.

The separation of body (i.e., matter) and mind was thoroughly cemented into Western culture with the seventeenth-century philosophy of Rene Descartes—matter became the province of science and mind (I include "mindset" here), that of religion and spirituality in general.

Gradually too the ancient natural remedies that served diverse populations around the planet for eons gave way to scientific "advances" of technologically manufactured, synthetic and derivative compounds devoid of the vital energy necessary to sustain vibrant life. Don't get me wrong; many of today's pharmaceutical "miracle drugs" save or prolong the lives of those who would perish without them—but at what cost?

Doctors, shamans, medicine men, and the like have always been held in high esteem by the societies and communities they serve; so much so that we have placed MDs on a pedestal, which is potentially problematic enough for the patient from a self-esteem standpoint, especially considering many doctors' lack of bedside manner. But the worst of it is that in so doing, we abdicate taking responsibility for our own health and well-being by deferring to someone outside ourselves to whom we hand over power and control.

With the founding of the American Medical Association (AMA) in the mid-nineteenth century, both as a regulatory body and advocacy organization, a doctor's position and stature became well established as a top-tier profession and career choice commanding respect and the potential of significant income.

Let me be clear. I am not throwing the baby out with the bathwater. Physicians save lives. And the degree of schooling and specialty required to diagnose, treat, and eradicate many types of disease is staggering! At the same time, the profession is plagued by the perception that pharmaceuticals and surgery drive treatment no matter what, and that the doctor always knows best what the patient needs, often without consulting the patient as to his or her lifestyle choices that are the root cause of the symptoms exhibited.

Enter Dr. Davisson Edmond, a board-certified medical doctor with a specialty in family medicine, who understands full-well that a patient's healing and well-being must involve the patients—their mindset, choices, and commitment to wellness. A lifelong student of personal development and accountability, Dr. Edmond asserts, "We are all responsible for our own health. It's not only *physician heal thyself.* It's no less patient heal thyself as well," he says.

Dr. Edmond puts forth a triarchic and holistic model of the person that includes three core elements—mind, body, and spirit—of which the mind (or mindset) is primary if not determinative in dictating the course of one's life. On the premise that our inner world creates our outer world, and that we choose to be victim or victor, we are empowered to choose health over sickness, vitality over malaise, positive outcomes over negative ones.

"Your health is your wealth," Dr. Edmond says, "and your actions will determine your results, the outcomes of your life." It's the accumulation over time of right choices, one by one, that can uplift us to new heights of awareness and experience, or little errors in judgment that can drag us down to the pits of despair, illness, and failure. It's up to you!

The good news is, we can "hit the reset button," as Dr. Edmond calls it. As only about 5 percent of disease is genetic, we have enormous range, power, and capability to reduce the toxins in our inner and outer environments, to monitor our activity as well as what we ingest, and to clear away the noxious programs and conditioning driving our lifestyle that plague us like the worst contagions on the planet.

Dr. Davisson Edmond is a physician for our times! Bridging the expanse between conventional Western medicine and what I call the "alternative modalities of healing," often ancient in their origins, he represents the best of both worlds! The book is both conceptual and prescriptive, pushing the envelope of the mainstream medical paradigm and its protocols, while providing a blueprint for taking charge of your own health—how to fix and prevent the root causes of your ailments, not just treat symptoms.

This book is for doctors and other health and wellness professionals who want to expand their vision of what constitutes healing; and it is written for laypersons as well who want a better quality of life knowing they have the reins to take it anywhere they wish.

Dr. James Alvino, PhD
Independent Business Coach
JT Foxx Organization

ACKNOWLEDGMENTS

I would like to express special thanks to my mentor, JT Foxx, as well as my coach, Jim Alvino, who encouraged and guided me through writing this book.

CHAPTER 1

Your Health Is Your Wealth

What do I mean by this?

Wealth has always been equated to material possessions, bank accounts, and levels of influence, but in the grand scheme of things, you can have all the fortune in the world and have it not amount to *anything* because you do not have the health to enjoy it. It is important to ask ourselves, *What's the point of having all the wealth in the world if I don't have my health?*

Exactly my thoughts! It is accurate for me to say that my health is my only wealth. Many rich and famous people have died prematurely, some in their prime, such as Steve Jobs and Patrick Swayze, leaving behind fortune and fame. In the end, all their wealth did not save them. I'm certain they would've traded it all for a long and healthy life.

In everything we do, it is imperative we make sure our health comes first. It should be the center of attention, the one nonnegotiable in everyday life. Strong health is the foundation of any responsible living, the only assurance we can give ourselves, our children, and

1

our families. Once we have our health, we can conquer anything. With great health, we can be productive beyond measure.

Being a physician, I know without a shadow of a doubt that being healthy is the only thing that matters. It is our most precious possession—our "wealth."

This year has been a challenging one, with a colossal financial crisis triggered by a minuscule virus, COVID-19. Arguably not the deadliest virus we have encountered. It has created such fear and panic that the whole world went on massive lockdown, resulting in one of the greatest financial and human crises of the century. Millions lost their jobs because of the fear of losing their lives. In my professional and personal observation, the virus is not the cause, but the flagrant precarious state of our personal and collective health is.

Growing up in Haiti, my lifestyle was different from when I first lived in the states. I was always playing outside, eating unprocessed food, and playing different sports with family and friends in the neighborhood. I was always happy. The rare moments I was unhappy were usually because I got into trouble with my mother. I remember seldom being sick.

I have been working out religiously in the gym since I was fourteen and always maintained a great physical shape, which powered me through the six grueling years of medical school. After I graduated, I came to the states to attend residency, and during those three years I gained more than pounds. I can say those were the most challenging and distraught years of my journey. The hundred-plus hours a week workload, emotional and physical stress, the lack of time to exercise, and not eating a nutritious diet spiraled me into severe depression and fatigue with a sense of hopelessness and being out of control.

How I survived residency is still a mystery to me. But shortly after finishing, I became somewhat aware of the difference between my quality of life, well-being, and joy before I lost my health. In a way it was a price to pay. At that time I realized that no amount of money or credentials were worth one's health.

Three Core Philosophies

Mindset Is Everything

Mindset is about your awareness, your presence of mind. I compare it to software powering the manifestations in our lives, manifestations are the realities we create with our state of mind, our thoughts, we are where we are in life because of how we've felt and acted upon those feelings. Most of us run on old "software" stored in our subconscious mind. We execute the same commands and get the same results over and over. No wonder we feel so powerless and desperate at times, unable to feel any different or produce any different reality than the ones to which we have become accustomed.

it took me decades to understand that concept. Our mindset, awareness in the mind, determines where our focus and energy in life go, so it determines what we manifest in our lives. That's why I say it all starts there; to be able to will our awareness in the mind we need to first acquire that insight either by inspiration or influence. That's why it is important to surround ourselves with the right people. Then we need to develop the concentration and willpower to keep awareness locked down on what we want to realize and manifest into existence.

In my quest for understanding the mind and its inner working, I have spent the past few years reading different authors, studying and practicing different schools of thought and methodologies. Some are more pertinent than others, but I have come to the realization that although numerous, it all came to the same conclusion: mindset is the primary driver of all existence. Either you realize it or not, the consciousness or unconsciousness of it.

My understanding of consciousness is that without it, we wouldn't have the dignity of choice we have as human beings. A quality— or imperfection, depending on how we want to see it. Because as a race we can decide what action to take or not. We have preferences that often lead to prejudices, and it overrides our instinct. Instinct is the default programming of every animal, nature itself, the modus operandi, which assures that every life form as we know them work in harmony, intertwined for the greater good. Only one life form is exempt: humankind.

One of my mentors once said, "All life forms strive to the best of their ability, except human beings. How tall can a tree get? As tall as he can." But in the end, the tree can only be a tree no matter how tall it can get. Human potential is limitless. We are capable of manifesting destruction and calamity upon ourselves and others by tapping into our lowest selves, such as genocide, war, and poverty, to mention a few. And we are capable of God-like deeds, such as bringing hope to others, peace, entering outer space, and healing the sick when we tap into our higher selves.

As I explored the domain of mindset, I came to the realization that most of us are far from being conscious; we operate at a subconscious level. A lot of ink has been poured on the subject of subconscious versus conscious. Dr. Joe Dispenza, whose work fascinates me, teaches that mind is nothing but matter and energy. Once we become conscious of that, we can create our reality from within and break free of the past programming of the subconscious, escaping the Newtonian world of cause and effect to the quantum physic of "causing an effect." Dr. Hew Len and Dr. Joe Vitale follow the Ho'Oponopono philosophy, a Hawaiian practice of reconciliation and forgiveness, which focuses more on rehabbing and cleaning the subconscious mind when it manifests in our lives by constantly "cleaning" by repeating a few words (such as I love you, I'm sorry, please forgive me, and thank you).

In the end it all comes to the same conclusion: unless we become aware of the inner workings between the conscious and subconscious minds, we are bound to wander endlessly in our journey called life without ever reaching our destination—fulfillment and self-actualization.

The Goal of Consciousness Health Is to Overcome Dissociation

Conscious health is a constant balance between body, mind, and spirit. We can't dissociate the three. Just like our hearts beat, we breathe in order to sustain life, and so is the constant balance between a healthy mind and healthy spirit in a healthy body. In order to produce any change in our lives, the mind and body have to be in alignment, not in opposition—we have to feel how we think. The great majority of the people I encounter in my practice and life are usually in a dissociative state. A state where there is no awareness of the need for mind, body and spirit to be nurtured and connected. Ancient civilizations had a better understanding of the importance of such, our current society not so much. We have been thought to regard the body as separated from the mind and the spirit. Therefore, relegated to different disciplines, you see the doctor for the body, religion caters to the spirit, the mind is usually forgotten. We need to be mindful of that crucial concept, we need to understand that we have the power and responsibility to attend to all three. The greater the dissociation, the more severe their ailments tend to be for example, metabolic diseases such as diabetes and maladaptive disorders such as depression and anxiety.

We primarily cause our own reality through deeply rooted subconscious programs and memories, even at the cellular level. We have permitted the external world and our experiences to dictate our view of the *now*, never breaking the habit of being ourselves. Dr. Joe Dispenza discussed this well in his book *Breaking the Habit of Being Yourself*. We are who we are now because of the things that have happened to us in the past, that's what we need to break ties with. To see, do and be different than we have thus far we need to change who we are. We have mentally and chemically created an automated self, a personality, existing like a recorded loop of our past but never creating.

Most of us have not been awakened. The memories and conditioning programs residing in the subconscious mind run our day-to-day lives, often creating a dull monotony. We may at times have a brief Satori moment (a deep, abiding insight in which someone sees and understands the true nature of the universe and of reality itself). We become conscious of the conundrum and override our subconscious-created selves—our personalities—and in that moment we feel great and centered; we become conscious of our infinite potential to weave a limitless reality.

Your Actions Determine Your Results

Change doesn't occur without action—the right action. Without action, there is no manifestation, no results, no transformation. It begins at the level of mindset, consciousness. From the neocortex down to the cerebellum, the appropriate mindset triggers our genes to release chemicals (such as neurotransmitters, hormones, and proteins) responsible for our physical experiences and our ultimate personality, which define our reality. Either we look at it from a physiological point of view or through the lens of quantum (the observer effect) change requiring consciousness in action.

This twenty-first century, the era of knowledge, has seen the highest numbers of metabolic, maladaptive diseases and poverty when the how-tos and the dos and don'ts are so readily available. Never before have we depended so much on our external stimuli to navigate our day-to-day lives (there's an app for everything). Instead of being creators causing effect on the outer world, we have surrendered to the predictable and comfortable preset self of the cause and effect Newtonian world dominated by the outer world (body, time, environment).

No matter the magnitude of change needed, it cannot be realized without action—most importantly the right action. "The journey of a thousand miles starts with a single step," says philosopher Lao Tzu. No great intentions will bring change unless acted upon.

I often say to my seven-year-old son that practice doesn't make perfect; practice makes permanent. Practice is taking action, but we all know, for example, if you practice the wrong swing in golf or the wrong form in tennis, you will never become good. To be able to manifest anything different in our lives, it is imperative to execute the right action consistently through mindset. Using our mindset to change our reality, from the inside out, is taking full responsibility.

"You must take personal responsibility. You cannot change the circumstances, the seasons, or the wind, but you can change yourself. That is something you have charge of. How you do one thing is how you do everything," says American entrepreneur, author, and motivational speaker, Jim Rohn.

Taking the right action, personal responsibility, is also the great divider, the difference maker, the gap between those who succeed and those who fail.

"People on the success curve live a life of full responsibility for who they are, where they are, and everything that happens to them," says entrepreneur Jeff Olson. Speaking of success, he adds, "Successful people do what unsuccessful people are unwilling to do."

You Have the Power to Change

We have the power to change our current reality, according to three core philosophies: health is your wealth, mindset is everything, and right action gets results. You and I are not mere passive recipients of whatever fate hands us; once woken, we can become active shapers of our ideal health and overall lives.

My Purpose in Writing This Book

My primary objective is to bring the concept of conscious health to my peers. People come to health-care professionals to nurture them back to health. It is time that we stop making a dissociation between mind, body, and spirit when it comes to health. We need one important principle, when it comes to health, an approach of the individual as a whole: mind, body, and spirit. It is time that we get back on track, back on the path set by Hippocrates, who argued that disease was not a punishment inflicted by the gods but rather the product of environmental factors, diet, and living habits.

Modern medicine has made great leaps in technology and treatments, and we are grateful for many of those, but treatment has become our sole focus and obsession, like mad scientists. We have neglected our primary duty, prevention—do no harm. We diagnose primarily to come up with the question, "How do I treat this?" instead of "Why is this happening?" Which leads us to prescribe a drug to palliate the effect, not to reverse the cause of a disease, a drug with multiple deleterious side effects at times—even death.

No wonder, during an on-stage interview with Dr. Phil at the 2019 Mega Success Event in Los Angeles, where I asked him why he thought, despite it being proven that an ounce of prevention was worth more than a pound of cure, that we still try to treat diseases after the fact rather than before. He answered that it is because prevention doesn't make our current pharmaceutical-driven health-care system any money. Imagine for a moment the financial impact eradicating most cases of diabetes, hypertension, and cancer would have on Big Pharma by just bringing awareness to people that living responsibly can positively impact their overall health and well-being.

I'm not anti-pharmaceutical, nor anti-progress in the field of medicine. I prescribe medications and use various advanced technologies to help my patients in my day-to-day practice. We are able to treat infectious and communicable diseases people were dying from a few decades ago. We are basically able to perform miracles at times because of the advanced techniques and gadgets we now have at our disposal when it comes to surgery, trauma, and neonatology, to mention a few.

Davisson Edmond, M.D.

I see myself as the bridge between conventional and conscious medicine with a focus on mindset as the foundation to manifest great health and quality of life from within similar to the observer effect in quantum laws. It's different from integrative medicine, which neither rejects conventional medicine nor accepts alternative modalities uncritically.

My relentless quest and dedication to personal development the last five years have led me to my current perspective. The ability to become our best selves, to manifest the reality we pursue in our health and overall lives already lies within us. We need to gain awareness of our limitless potential, divorce the victimhood mentality and dogmas, commit to the right action, and harness our innate power. We need to become centered in the self.

CHAPTER 2

We Are Not Victims

Considering what we have discussed so far, we must realize we are 100 percent responsible for our lives. We are not victims of circumstance, we are subconsciously the perpetrators. It is time that we realize our limitless conscious potential and take whole responsibility for how our lives and the lives of those around us unfold.

What about Genetics and the Environment?

The field of genetics is fascinating. It is amazing to imagine that all the information necessary to express every detail of living beings, from their physical attributes to their physiological functions and even their lifespans, is encrypted in a unique sequence, DNA.

How does the genome work? It was thought that the gene is simple information that codes for a particular feature, either physical or physiological, essential to express a specific characteristic, trait, or ability, even determining our predisposition to certain diseases and infections. But recent studies have shown that our DNA, genome, is influenced greatly by various extrinsic factors, such as environment, nutrition, and thought (mindset).

Epigenetics tells us a lot more about this. It is the study of the effect of environment and nutrition on overall health. The food we ingest, the level of pollution in the environment, and the presence or absence of the right bacteria or microbe have a big impact on gene activation or deactivation.

Fewer than 5 percent of diseases are genetic in nature, such as cystic fibrosis, Tay-Sachs disease, or Down syndrome. The other 95 percent of the diseases we are plagued with are a direct results of genes' improper activation or inhibition. We are seldom victims of diseases; they are a direct translation of our own actions or inactions in the manner in which we live, eat, and think.

That is great news! Knowing this allows us to establish that the majority of our ailments are fully reversible. They are the results of faulty transcription, not faulty genes, borne of our own doing. In many cases we are able to hit the reset button!

Take Full Responsibility

We live during a time where personal responsibility is rare. We have relinquished control because we are afraid of the outcome. We would rather suffer the consequences of someone's else decision than face our own.

I used to have the same phobia: *What if?* Until I realized that avoiding responsibility for my life always resulted in frustration. I began to assume responsibility, to get out of my comfort zone, to accept the possibility of failure as the price to pay to succeed. In the end it was easier to ingest failure at my own hand because it became a learning experience, a step closer to my objective instead of the sterile frustrations I have experienced. Taking responsibility is the only way to growth, and it's the gateway to changing one's mindset.

Nothing Is Permanent

Nothing in this experience called life is permanent, and health conditions are no exception. The majority of us remember how life, our health in particular, was uneventful and easygoing until we reached a certain age, and then everything changed. Our weight became a problem, we lacked energy, and maladaptive behaviors emerged. How did this happened? Our luck ran out!

Although this honeymoon period has gotten shorter the last two decades, with a higher prevalence of metabolic and behavioral illnesses occurring much sooner, the fact remains that nothing is permanent. Diabetes, hypertension, depression, anxiety, and cancer, for example, are transient conditions. They should be regarded as such, the focus placed on reestablishing a balanced life through the perfect mindset, conscious nutrition, and physical discipline in order to reverse them. Hit the reset button.

What Is Mindset?

Mindset is a learned behavior. It is who we are, our personalities. Not all mindset is healthy; some behaviors cause physical ailments because of the physiological changes they orchestrate. The mind is the live expression of the brain, like the melody we hear at a recital is the live expression of the instrument performing in a specific sequence.

Just like the sequence and manner in which striking an instrument determines the melody being played, the way we fire our brain consistently to a certain stimulus determines our mindset.

The brain, like a maestro, is responsible for homeostasis, which is basically the unconscious self. The self is the default system we run the majority of the time to interact with or interpret the basic stimuli of our day-to-day lives: time, body, and environment. The brain achieves this by firing the appropriate neuro-nets, which release the appropriate neurotransmitter and peptides in order to activate either our sympathetic or parasympathetic nervous systems—survival or growth.

Survival Emotions versus Wellness Emotions

The body calls upon the sympathetic nervous system when it comes to survival. This is the flight or fight mode, and the focus is on preparing the body for any current or perceived threats. Survival mode prioritizes the physiological processes needed for preservation, because existence is at stake: fear, anger, depression, anxiety, and hatred are expressions of a survival mindset.

Nurturing and growth are the drivers of wellness, and the body calls upon the parasympathetic nervous system. This is the law and order mode, and the focus is on the vital functions and processes necessary to maintain order and growth for the long run. The result is a centered self: energetic, positive, optimistic, joyous, creative, and inspired mindset.

CHAPTER 3

We Can Restore and Reset

As we discussed earlier, nothing is permanent; change has always been intrinsic to life, but life itself has an identity, a default mode. For so long we have been taken on a nonsensical ride when it comes to our health and well-being. We have sometimes been forced into a fictional world of recommendations and guidelines that serves the interest of many, except ours. We have inherited a paradigm shift where biased epidemiological studies are held for proof of unquestionable truth, and we have thus distanced ourselves from the fundamentals of life. We are so confused by the constant bombardment of misleading data that even the results we experience are not questioned. The old adage "the proof is in the pudding" doesn't even trigger our superior intelligence to question the proceedings.

Nonetheless, the capacity to reset our health and let how genetics programming express the best version of ourselves is as simple as flipping a switch, as long as we know such a switch exits. My mission is to make you aware of such and help guide you through this conundrum, to hit the reset button—we all have that ability; it's an implicit characteristic of our humanity.

15

Mind, Body, and Spirit

Mind, body, and spirit form the tripod of our essence; not to be dissociated or isolated, since we can't have a complete reset without reforming this trinity as one unit. The cartesian mind-body dualism approach of the seventeenth century continues to have a stronghold on our perception and quest of a balanced well-being far into this twenty-first century, but we will discover in the course of this book that this dualism is a hindrance to our ultimate quest.

Although it is undeniable that we all possess the inner workings to achieve optimum health through our genetics, it is not possible without the right choices, the right actions.

CHAPTER 4

How to Restore and Reset

Mens Sana In Corpore Sano

The first step to changing anything is self-awareness, which is imperative in changing one's life and overall health. Awareness starts in the mind, in an inner intelligence that guides us in our most subconscious states at times, like a gut feeling; that awareness of self in the mind can at times happen randomly, without any extrinsic stimuli; other times in can be triggered by a pivotal moment in our lives: either an event that forces us to take inventory of our current situation or an individual whose life or philosophy shed light on a path we've always felt attracted to. It has been the case for me on many occasions. Mindset is everything. It is the compass to any conscious destination, because without that guide or awareness we can achieve no fulfilling state of being. Sane health starts with a sane mindset—*mens sana in corpore sano*, which roughly translated from the Latin means "a healthy mind in a healthy body."

Our first commitment is to self-awareness and self-development. This is key to the next level up, and we owe it to ourselves and the world. Many of us go to our graves with our greatness and potential contributions to this world buried inside us for many reasons: our limiting associations, the suppressive dogmas of the society we live in, the fears embedded in us by our experiences, and the beliefs we hold true.

Committing to the right actions is the next concomitant step required; as discussed previously, this step is crucial in moving the needle forward. Great intentions have rarely produced any real change other than frustration and anguish in the end; many make resolutions every New Year's Eve to change their lives, but few succeed because of their inaction.

To reset my health, I had to start by taking inventory of my current health. I weighed more than 250 pounds, almost sixty pounds heavier than my ideal; I couldn't even make it through the first minute of the Beachbody Insanity program fit test without being completely gassed. I had a problem on my hands, one that could only spiral out of control with disastrous consequences down the road. However painful was that assessment and realization, it was necessary in order for me to change direction.

I'm asking you now to make the same assessment of your current health. Be honest and loving with yourself—this is not about shaming anyone or putting anyone down, it is about awareness of your potential—about living your best self, creating your optimal life.

I then had to identify the proper actions I need to take in order to change the course of my health, with the help of many proven blueprints already established, such as calorie restriction, proper nutrition and supplementation, physical activities, and mindfulness.

We all go on a journey to achieve our best form at different stages in our lives, so the approach has to be individualized in order to arrive at our desired outcome. We must constantly calculate and adjust our trajectory, so we continually track our actions and results. In order to make the adjustments necessary to obtain your goals, you have to foster consistency in your methods.

Mind, body, and spirit have to be in perfect alignment, in perfect congruence once more for us to be able to truly manifest our pure form. We have to become aware to change the mindset—the compass we wave to condition the body though the right nutrition and physical disciplines to house the bright flame of the mind, which allow us to forge healthy emotions and character: our spirit.

CHAPTER 5

Scripts for Changing and Maintaining a Positive Lifestyle

Mind

Meditation is one of the best tools we can use to gain awareness in the mind and change our mindset. I have learned the complexity of this skill from different masters, including guru Dandapani and Dr. Joe Dispenza. I ultimately developed my own practice in meditation based on my own inner truth. Many see meditation as a way to empty one's mind, a method to silence the incessant monologue playing in our heads, a way to relieve our stress. Meditation is a meeting with the higher self; it is about taking inventory of our "operating system"—the subconscious—and making necessary updates from within. Meditation is an engaging and focused process that directs your energy, vibration, and frequency to the reality you seek to manifest. Everything is energy, all animated and unanimated beings are pure energy with a vibration and frequency; to connect with anything therefore is a matter of aligning with the energy, frequency and vibration of what we desire.

The majority of us living in highly developed countries like the United States are workaholics, although most are really stagnating on all levels despite the unbelievable number of hours devoted to work or other related activities. There's little to no time for rejuvenation—no idling time. To be always doing something is such a pervasive act in our society that most would describe any downtime as being bored, not realizing that without downtime there's no chance for a reset.

I've found it crucial for my health to create downtimes where I don't do anything but take in the marvelous ride life is. During these periods I enjoy traveling with my family and friends, I let my imagination and mind run wild, I set free all my senses, and I open myself to new experiences; just like a sponge, I soak up the essence of this world. This creates a life balance for me that some would argue doesn't exist; that is, if you see balance as something static, but nothing is ever static in this universe; all and everything is dynamic and sequential. Nature is the best teacher in that regard.

Personal development is another tool to forging the right mindset, although I acknowledge the existence of an inner intelligence along with some level of inherited preset subconscious programs passed down by our ancestors, where experience is the ultimate character builder. We can acquire that experience through our own trials and errors or those of others who have set sail before us on the same quest. I'm constantly reading and learning from others in my fields of interest, and then I commit to the right actions.

"Learning is the beginning of wealth. It is the beginning of health. Learning is the beginning of spirituality. Searching and learning is where the miracle process all begins," says Jim Rohn.

Positive self-talk and affirmations—"I am"—are the most powerful words one can ever think or voice because they prophesize one's state of being. Beware of what comes after those two words! We tend to identify with our feeling and circumstances by saying things like, "I'm depressed," "I'm poor," or "I'm nobody," not realizing the boundaries and limitations we set for ourselves. We are limitless beings—until we decide to identify with a particular state that does not elevate our being. I use affirmations on a daily basis, phrases such as, "I'm healthy," and "I'm wealthy," with an elevated emotion during my meditations and randomly during the day. It tunes me into the quantum field just like tuning your TV to the desired channel.

Nikola Tesla said, "If you wish to understand the Universe think of energy, frequency and vibration."

Our doubts and inability to formulate superior self-thoughts and mindsets have taken us off our true path because our energy (focus), frequency, and vibration have been set on the wrong wavelength.

Body

Nutrition is the foundation for a healthy body, but we have strayed from that concept in our westernized lifestyle. Food has become another commodity, heavily commercialized, manufactured to satisfy our addictions and lower emotions, not for the needs of our body. The resulting effects of such culture is more than evident in all aspect of our lives, but the problem is very much ignored. We live in a world heavily regulated by laws, particularly when it comes to health care. Therefore, why is the main culprit poisoning our body on such a laissez-faire policy? If you ask me,

I would say that dealing with the problem, regulating nutrition, would not benefit the status quo; such regulations would cause a disastrous financial domino effect for our current handlers (Big Pharma, food corporations, and the like).

We have been pitched so many different diets as healthy and best for us: vegan, low carb, keto, Mediterranean, and Miami Beach to name a few, but the fundamentals remain that the body needs certain nutrients and not all are compatible with our specific genetics. I have read about, researched, and experimented with many of those diets; I now understand a few universal fundamentals: source/origin, compatibility, toxins, or nutrients.

When it comes to source/origin, the fewest processes between us and our food the better. I shop for goods that are certified organic, grass fed, contain no hormones or antibiotics, cage free, and have no artificial ingredients. Most of the time we have no awareness of the effect the foods we ingest have on our well-being. I love my vegan friends, but plants themselves are the undisputed number-one pesticide and harmful chemical makers, such as sulforaphane, isothiocyanate, and oxalate, that is their main mechanism of defense and ingesting them causes short- and long-term complications to their aggressors, including gastrointestinal, musculoskeletal, immunological, and neurological ailments, some currently being studied for possible carcinogenic effects. The focus should be on what the nutrients being offered are, preferably not in a Trojan horse fashion. Our digestive tracts, microbiomes, and genetics are not compatible with all that we shove in—because our bodies compensate, adjust, and don't pass for acceptance.

Nowadays, lots of toxins in our diet along with their numerous short- and long-term deleterious effects on our body have been well studied. Why are they still being marketed and forced upon us? But just like the slogan "Cheerios help lower your cholesterol" have many of my cardiac and metabolic disease sufferers indulge in a large bowl of Cheerios with A1 beta-casein milk from cows injected with bovine somatotropin (bST)—despite the fact it has not produced any impactful change in the natural progression of their conditions, simply because we have been conditioned to comply—at times blindly—to a societal consciousness. Whereas in reality, causality has never been established between dietary cholesterol and vascular and other metabolic diseases.

The so-called studies used to advance agendas such as the low-fat diet like the epic Framingham study are all epidemiological/observational studies riddled with different biases that were also ignored. These epidemiological studies can only establish correlation at best, not causation. Most use such studies as "scientific proof" to spawn different health and nutritional guidelines, including medications such as statins for lowering cholesterol (an innocent on death row) even when scientifically it has been shown that statins don't lower risk of MI/CVA (myocardial infarction and cerebrovascular accident) in secondary prevention by lowering cholesterol, they do so apparently by reducing inflammation.

It's hard to understand that despite the rate our estimated thirty trillions cells are being replaced and repaired, with new neuronal pathways being established, the cell membranes biodynamic needs, steroid hormones needed for stress response, and other vital functions, the lower our total cholesterol and LDL levels are the better off we are, when they are both crucial to these cited processes. Taking all this into consideration and the fact that our bodies produce the equivalent of three to six egg yolks in cholesterol a day versus the misleading mechanism of action of statins and their side effects like weight gain, increased chance for diabetes, poor sleep, poor cognition, neuropathy, musculoskeletal discomfort, and behavioral changes such as increased irritability and aggression. All that to just reduce inflammation and prevent LDL from getting stuck into my arterial walls regardless of the number of LDL—taking into consideration the "LDL cholesterol paradox," which makes me acknowledge more and more the response-to-retention hypothesis. Wouldn't it make more sense to focus on what's causing the inflammation in the first place, considering it is the omnipresent factor in most disease processes including CAD (coronary artery disease), diabetes, hypertension, autoimmune disease, obesity, and cancer, to name a few?

I know, firsthand, now that an anti-inflammatory diet and lifestyle are key to reversing and preventing many of the ailments we become afflicted with, because I've personally adopted many of the "healthy" and organization-endorsed diets, such as whole grain, or bountiful amounts of fruits and vegetables, only to learn the truth later at the expense of my own ailments and discomforts after adopting those recommendations about things like lectins, isothiocyanates, oxalates, sulforaphanes, fructose (the main sugar in fruits), and GMOs (genetically modified foods). Like many, I bought into the social consciousness at first and ignored my disillusion for a while. I focused on the few said benefits although the drawbacks were evident until I got fed up and unplugged from the matrix to search for the missing piece: results.

I was flabbergasted to realize that many doctors and scientists have taken their blindfolds off a long time ago and had written about the wrongs of our industry and consumer-driven diet and health recommendations; they researched through personal experimentation, careful examination of previous studies and their biases, and results from other subjects and patients. Boosted by my own results, I started, in my private practice, to make changes in the sterile and generic recommendations of the mainstream to recommending a more DIY—do-it-yourself—conscious way, starting with a clean and more compatible nutrition to maximize our body's capabilities and potential. The cognitive dissonance and skepticism from most of my patients was not surprising and were well understood on my part.

Nonetheless, I couldn't in good conscience and ethics not bring it to their awareness. The ones who trusted me were in search of a change to the status quo, an end to their suffering and the powerless feeling of having to rely on an armful of medications and ineffective regimes in hope of prolonging a life of poor quality at best; but they didn't see a way out beside the hope that tomorrow could finally be the day they sudden see the so-long-awaited benefits. Those brave ones have seen results that include reversal of their diabetes, high blood pressure, rheumatoid arthritis, fibromyalgia, chronic pain, morbid obesity, chronic pain, depression, and anxiety, among other conditions; but nothing was worth more than the majority of them gradually being able to come off all or most of their medications while maintaining the afflictions away and enjoying a superior quality of life. They have discovered the benefits of conscious health and responsible living.

Sleep

Most of us do not need a reminder on the importance of sleep on our well-being. It is the most crucial part of recovery, growth, and wellness. The amount needed for optimal results vary from one individual to another depending on their level of physical and mental strain. For example, babies sleep most of the day, on average eighteen to twenty hours, because they are going through a tremendous growth and developmental phase; adolescents and teenagers require about ten hours on average, although these days it is about seven hours because of all the addictive stimuli they are subject to. And we wonder why so many teenagers face depression and other behavioral afflictions.

Most adults should thrive on an average of seven hours sleep a day; fewer than five hours a day is detrimental to optimum health. I have suffered firsthand the effects of sleep deprivation throughout my career as a physician, accumulating years of fewer than thirty hours a week, sometimes even fewer than twenty; those effects were mood and behavioral disorders, metabolic syndrome, obesity, low self-esteem, personal failures, and poor mindset while saving others' lives and nurturing them to health. In case you didn't know, this is the reality of most doctors when it comes to sleep and its deleterious effects on their lives. Next time you have access to a physician, be mindful of that individual who is caring for you, and appreciate their sacrifices; it's their calling.

The last couple of years I have committed myself to a better sleep schedule, six hours on average, and it has been a game changer for me on so many levels: better mindset with centered focus, discipline, meaningful work, and resiliency, although I had to say no to many things and responsibilities that were not necessary in the end in order for me to gain a consistent and beneficial sleep schedule.

I recommend that everyone establish a set time to go to bed and to wake up in the morning, depending on their life schedule and age. I'm a ten p.m. to five a.m. kind of guy. It's preferable to keep a cool temperature in the bedroom, below sixty-eight degrees, use dark drapes or a blackout curtain to keep the room dark, and it's best to keep electronic and blue light devices out of the bedroom. If you need your cell phone as an alarm, plug it in the bathroom. The old radio clock at the bedside is a better option in my opinion. When your alarm goes off, don't snooze.

Get up and seize the day. I sometimes use the "five-second rule" (from his book *The 5-Second Rule* by Mel Robbins), which says if you have an instinct to act on a goal, you must physically move within five seconds or your brain will kill it. The moment you feel an instinct or a desire to act on a goal or a commitment, do it. This is a great personal development book, by the way. I recommend you read it.

Hormesis is defined by toxicologists as a biphasic dose response to an environmental agent with a low-dose stimulation showing beneficial effects and a high-dose stimulation showing inhibitory or toxic effects. Many wellness and fitness aficionados know about the benefits of hormesis. Heat and cold exposure is a good example of how low gradual exposure to high and low temperatures can be beneficial to the body and our overall well-being.

Since humans first ate from the tree of knowledge, their descent from being elevated creatures started. Our knowledge brought us the comforts we are used to and depend on, and we have in a way rebelled against nature's guidance and wisdom by creating our own realities—for example, constant climate control, manipulation and control of our food supply all year long, and infecting and disrupting the ecosystem. That has given us the false pretense of being the ultimate human being because of our achievements, whereas it is the absolute opposite; by sheltering ourselves and overriding nature's challenges, we have actually created a weaker human being.

I practice heat and cold exposure on a regular basis. I use an infrared sauna at home for my heat exposure about three or four times a day. I alternate days and do my ten-minute cold plunge. I usually spend about thirty or forty minutes in the sauna to a max temperature of 142 degree. I sometimes meditate a second time in the day or reflect on something that stimulates my higher self.

The benefits of heat exposure, the infrared sauna in particular, are immeasurable. Some of these benefits include antiaging, helping detox heavy metals and toxins, increasing longevity, improving insulin sensitivity, boosting our immune system, and lowering the risks of metabolic diseases. It is also a way for me to relax and empty my mind and do some yoga and other functional exercises.

Cold exposure would be my favorite, if there were such thing, because it is the most challenging to me. Immersing yourself, free will, neck deep into fifty-degree water for several minutes is not most people's idea of healthy; the usual reaction I get is, "Are you crazy?" But I never felt better in my life since adding cold exposure to my wellness regimen. The metabolic, anti-inflammatory, and psychological benefits were almost instantaneous; within a month of daily cold showers, I've noticed an increase in energy and clarity of mind throughout the day. By ninety days I have dropped about fifteen pounds along with 2 percent body fat, and my joints and muscles recover faster with less pain, reducing the number of visits to my massage therapist.

In general, cold exposure helps increase our percentage of brown fat, increases insulin sensitivity, reduces proinflammatory interleukins, slows down the aging process, and strengthens the immune system. It also has many psychological effects, including increased resilience, decisiveness, and helping manage depression and anxiety.

Spirit

Attending to the spiritual aspect of our being is of upmost importance in our quest for conscious health. Spirituality encompasses some of the timeless enigmas of our existence: Is there a Supreme Creator of all life? Who am I? Why am I here? What is this life about? What is evil and good? What is after death? Religions and doctrines have attempted to answer many of those existential questions, but in my experience most have not helped us understand that we are one with the answers we seek; we have become unconscious of our divinity. Humankind has led himself and herself to believe that creation is outside of our reach, despite all the evidence that the world as he or she is experiencing it now is the product of each person's own thoughts and creativity; we have become so materialistic, so solid, that we have no recollection of the light and energy source that we are.

Similar to an intuition, a gut feeling, or sixth sense, we seek what I would compare to a transcendental consciousness, which is described as being awake with no object of consciousness. A state of being where the subject and the object are just one, interdependent and nonpermanent, a state of no-self and no-time, ever changing. We seek something greater than what have become, greater than our current dominant material form; we seek a way back to our higher conscious energy form; we seek the isness of all: God.

The moment we realize who we really are, the power within us, we can start manifesting the life experience we want. We are conscious energy, and everything around us is energy, the entire cosmos is; therefore, everything has a frequency and a vibration, just like Tesla enunciated, and to manifest anything we want in life, we have to broadcast the frequency and vibration of that which we wish to experience. The observer effect in quantum physics describes such phenomenon observing particles in the atom as observer bias.

We are a creative intelligence who has abdicated its sovereignty to its subjects and creation. The servant has become the master, and we need to become aware of that reversal of roles. We need to revert to a causing effects–enlightened spiritual state instead of the subconscious cause-and-effect purgatory state we are trapped in. We need to see the material world we have created as a reflection of our divinity and free ourselves from it.

Conscious health is the perfect balance of mind, body, and spirit well-being; it is about being whole. It can only be obtained through deliberate practice of awareness, focus, and discipline toward self-development and self-realization. It is the path of most resistance.

CHAPTER 6

Thrive and Grow

Once I gained awareness of my inner power and acknowledged the divine creator within, my life has never been the same. I no longer live in the world of uncertainty of causes and effects. I'm causing the desired effects in my life with the vibrational power of my thoughts as I prune away the thoughts that are not in alignment with the things I want to attract, like great health and the freedom wealth provides.

Demanding the highest standard of purity from ourselves, being a centered and harmonious self, is the path to thrive and grow. When we thrive and grow, we elevate ourselves and our reality, including everyone else's around us because of our interdependence. When we shine brighter, we light up the path for others, and we ignite their souls and strengthen our collective reality.

When we are healthy, everyone benefits from our elevated energy and emotional vibe. We can contribute to the collective wealth and well-being of our family, friends, and community; we can be a model of best mind, body, and spirit—the example of what's possible, a leader.

Many of us live lives of absolute limitation because of our ignorance of what is possible for us, and we are caught up in a world that deems our individual light, a world that stripped us of our self-reliance, most of us having traded our limitlessness for the comfort of false securities.

An awakened self is an enrichment for our family in many ways. Conscious health brings forth the best expression of our genetics potential, allowing us to pass down to our unborn children a fully functional operating system, like handing them a lit candle instead of just the candle. To our already-born children and our spouse, an awakened self could be the spark that ignites their own enlightenment, their guide to conscious health and self-realization.

Will I leave the world better than I found it? No one can achieve such; it would mean that the world could be summed up to one person's reality, the better one, whereas we all have our own realities, self-realizations to bring to fruition on this plane. But the majority are asleep at the wheel. My quest is not to be a savior, guru, or expert of any sort. I want to leave behind the irrefutable truth of my own self-realization as a beacon of light for those seeking the path within. Everything we yearn for: health, wealth, love, and joy are within us, but we have been led to look for them elsewhere. We all need someone or something to point out this absolute truth to us, to liberate us from our external chains, to bear witness to our inner creative power. That's my legacy.

CHAPTER 7

Conclusion

In summary, health is tridimensional and must be nurtured. Unfortunately, our current health-care system and societal consciousness are caught up in the transactional webs of symptom management instead of dissecting the root causes of our afflictions.

We are not victims of circumstances when it comes to our state of health. We are the perpetrators in the way we live, the foods we ingest, the thoughts we entertain, and the beliefs we hold to be true. Most of us are unconscious with a hands-off attitude when it comes to our well-being. We need to regain consciousness of the power we have over our health and well-being; we need to start living responsibly. Once we understand that nothing in this universe is permanent, the majority of our health conditions as well, and that we in charge are not victims, life becomes limitless.

The first and most crucial step is awareness, mindset; a positive mindset is the catalyst to our innate creativity. It is the key to manifesting the health, wealth, and overall life we desire. The power to do anything is already seeded within each one of us. We have lost our connection to it because we have ventured so far out from the Source, we have been distracted by too many shiny concepts and been betrayed by our own comfort. Our body and materialistic attachment have become our definition, the servant has become the master, and our willpower-consciousness has been silenced.

I cannot emphasize or stress the importance of awareness enough in this book because I know it to be the gateway to what we all seek: self-realization and fulfillment. I was fortunate enough in my journey to be introduced to great thinkers/mentors, such as Jim Rohn, Tony Robbins, Darren Hardy, Dr. Joe Vitale, Dr. Hew Len, Dr. Joe Dispenza, guru Dandapani, Dr. Wayne Dyer, Siddhartha Gautama, and Thich Nhat Hanh, among countless others who have helped awaken my conscious self.

Just like no one element of a car is the car and cannot perform as the car by itself, no one entity of our being can perform holistically without the congruent dynamism of all three entities: mind, body, and spirit. Examples of this holistic trinity can be found in many cultures and religions throughout our human history and quest for the Supreme Creator, God: Trinity of Hindu, Christianity, the Capitoline Triad of ancient Rome, and the Holy Trinity of Gods of ancient Greece, to name a few.

To reach this level of holistic balance requires a relentless commitment to self-awareness, self-development, taking right actions, self-discipline, and consistency. All of which demand a break from inertia, from our comfort zone. We all innately know that we are greater than our current circumstances, that we are powerful, and that's why we seek the "greater than self" factor but not realizing we are it, another reason most of us live lives of quiet desperation. You can't find something where it is not.

My pilgrimage to conscious health is one of courage and endurance—the courage to engage and embrace the unknown, the endurance to apply myself to the different disciplines necessary. I have learned different ways to nurture my mind, body, and spirit throughout my exciting journey and I've felt compelled to share it with you in this book. As a physician, son of Asclepius, I can only sing the praises of all the progress medicine has made in the last fifty years alone, but I also have to acknowledge that most of us physicians have lost sight of our craft. We have become institutional puppets following guidelines and treatments that promise to solve one problem in exchange for many more, even death.

We have shifted from helping others restore their health form an unbalanced, diseased, or damaged self, enabling or supporting their inner healing abilities, to attacking their bodies with chemicals (medications) as if they were defective themselves. It is time we put the emphasis back on the engineering marvel we human are, omnipotent, and when we acknowledge that everything we need to thrive is already within us, we can free ourselves from suffering like brushing dust off our shoulders, and paint the reality we desire on the blank canvas of our time on this level of life.

Throughout this journey of self-awareness and self-development I have learned the invaluable role of guidance and coaching. I also know how difficult it is to find right guidance and coaching when it comes to conscious health, and I want to continue to be that beacon for you. Follow on Facebook, IG or www. consciouslifehealth.com more.

ABOUT THE AUTHOR

Davisson Edmond was born on July 18, 1979, in Port-au-Prince, Haiti. Medicine was his first love from a young age, growing up with a nurse as a mother and uncles who were doctors. He was an accident-prone child and told himself he would one day he a doctor. When the time came to embark on the six-year journey through medical school, the decision was clear.

Once he graduated from medical school in October 2004, he moved to the United States and completed a residency program in family medicine at the University of Arkansas for Medical Sciences (UAMS).

He has run a private practice in the small town of Oxford, Alabama, for the past six years. He likes to travel the world with his family and friends and takes care of his mother and other relatives in Haiti. He's married to Marie, a southern belle, and they have an energetic eight-year-old son, Ethan.

He's a workaholic, fitness fanatic, health nut, and serial entrepreneur who is currently focused on sharing his knowledge in medicine and personal development to help others change their mindsets to achieve conscious health and manifest their desired realities.

Made in the USA
Las Vegas, NV
14 July 2021

26392744R00035